Guide to Healthy Primal Living

Lev Well

ISBN: 1533494002
ISBN-13: 978-1533494009

Contents

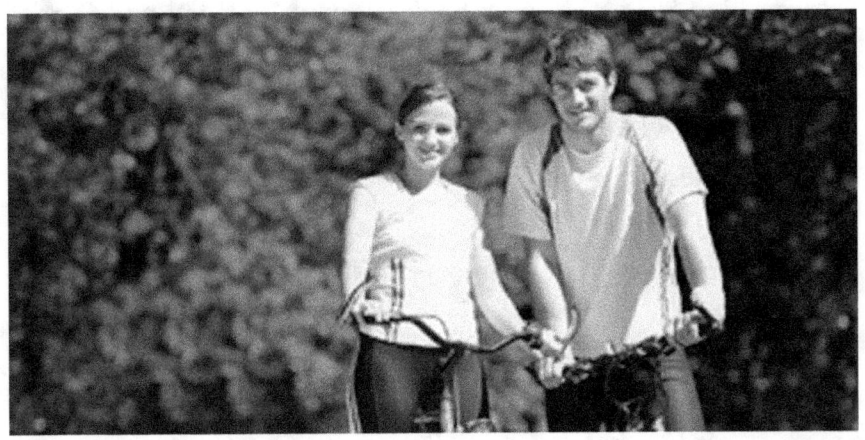

Chapter 1: Introduction – What is Primal Living? And Why You Should Care

If you've been keeping an eye on the fitness industry over the last few years, then you might have noticed some interesting changes in attitude.

Whereas fitness was once all about exercise machines, supplements and low-fat diets; today we're starting to go back to our roots.

Basically, we've found that these 'high tech' methods of losing weight, improving health and getting fitter just don't work as well as they should. And this really comes down to one simple truth: we can't do better than nature.

Today, health bloggers and thought leaders in the industry are preaching from a different book. Now we're being told to get outside more, to get sunlight, to swim in the cold water, to eat a balanced, natural diet and to train using our bodies and our environments.

And guess what? For the most part it's working!

99% of our health problems exist as a direct result of our modern lifestyles. That means processed foods that don't contain any nutrition. It means sitting at desks for 8 hours every day. It means constant chronic stress. And it means trying to cure everything with pills.

The solution isn't to add *more* unhealthy supplements, or to create foods with no sustenance. The solution is to take a step *backwards* and to look to the environment in which we first evolved. Experts agree that diabetes likely didn't exist (or at least was incredibly rare) only a few hundred years ago.

Obesity is higher than it has ever been.

We're living longer but our quality of lives are taking a hit. It seems we lost something important along the way.

Time to go back to basics and to get our health back!

A Quick Lesson in Evolution

The above statements are going to make an awful lot of sense to some people, while others might need a bit more convincing. Is the answer really as simple as 'not eating cake'? Can it really make that much difference whether you get your nutrition from an apple, or from a multivitamin?

The answer is a resounding yes. And it will affect more areas of your life than you can probably predict.

And the reason for this comes down to evolutionary biology. You probably have some basic idea of evolution but to bring you fully up to speed let's take a closer look at how it impacts with health.

Evolution comes down to natural selection. That is to say that the animals that survive are able to procreate and those that don't aren't. Thus, the DNA of the surviving animals gets passed on and iterated upon, whereas the 'failed' changes and mutations fall out of the runnings.

Over time, small mutations, individuals and epigenetics (more on this later) lead to species-wide changes.

All of the traits that we possess as a species therefore, exist because they were found to be the *optimal* traits that would help us to survive and thrive in our environments. That applies to our appearance, to our physical capabilities... even our psychology!

'Evolutionary psychology' is an entire school of psychology that seeks to explain our behaviour by looking at how it might have been 'selected for' during our evolution.

Altruism for example is adaptive because it allows us to ingratiate ourselves with groups and because it allows us to better survive as a group. Anger is adaptive because it helps us to protect our food sources, territory and social rank.

So far, so highschool science. We're going to go a lot deeper into the interplay between evolution and biology later on but for now, this is enough of a foundation to ensure you'll be able to follow the rest of what we're going to be looking at.

But now we need to think about the implications this has on our health.

And we need to start thinking about this the right way.

Some people will casually assume that natural foods are good for us because they've somehow been 'designed' for us. This is incorrect. The reality is that *our bodies* are designed *for* those foods.

We adapted to thrive on the foods we had available during our evolution because *that was what was available*.

We are *designed* to eat lots of fruits and vegetables, to eat lots of meats and to thrive on regular activity. This took millions of years.

But if you take us *out* of that environment, we're then forced to 'make do' with things we were never designed for.

We've been removed from our natural environment and as such, we cannot thrive. Think of it like taking a gold fish and putting it in the desert – hardly optimal and it's unlikely the goldfish is going to be able to thrive.

Or perhaps think of it like trying to drive a hatchback off road. It simply isn't *designed* to work under those conditions. It might still work and it might still be able to drive but it's not going to be as fast, as powerful or as healthy.

That's the situation *you're* in right now. And that's why we need to go back to basics and that's why we need to try and change our environment to be a little closer to the way we used to live.

A Caveat and Some Warnings

Before we go any further though, I first want to get something out of the way.

This is *not* a book about the Paleo diet. Yes, we will be exploring the Paleo diet and this is one of the biggest and most popular aspects of 'primal living'.

At the same time though, it is also not the answer to everything. Paleo is only one part of going primal and you also need to think about many other things – such as the way that you're going to exercise and the exposure you're getting to light and fresh air.

Moreover, the Paleo diet may also prove to be something of a modern fad in itself. The danger with the Paleo diet is that we may be 'throwing the baby out with the bath water'. We'll explore this in a little more detail but suffice to say that living primal and going back to your routes doesn't necessarily mean you have to give up milk and bread. You don't even necessarily have to give up multivitamins and supplements.

We'll learn a lot more later on. But suffice to say, things are going to get pretty interesting and this *isn't* just a book promoting a diet that happens to be popular right now…

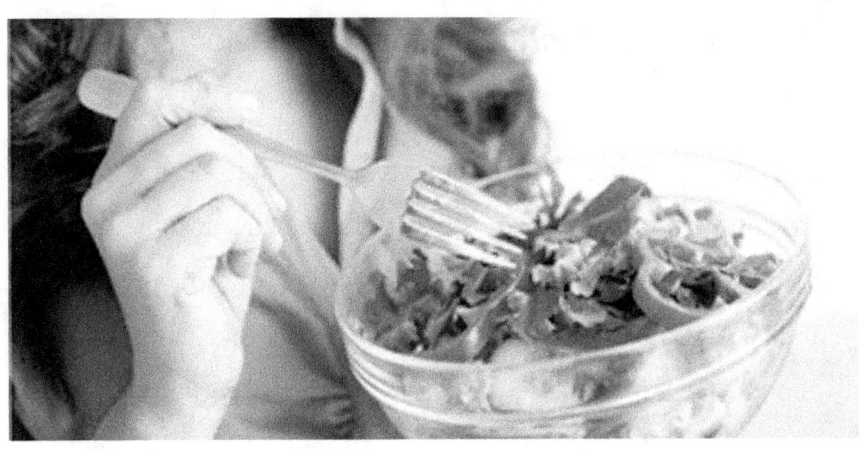

Chapter 2: Eating Primal

With all that said, a lot of you are probably coming into this expecting to learn about the Paleo diet. This is what many people will most associate with 'primal living' and so it makes sense rather to address the elephant in the room first.

What is the Paleo diet?

What's the general idea behind it?

Does it work?

Which elements should you adopt or ignore?

Let's answer all of those things…

A Basic Introduction to the Paleo Diet

The main concept behind the Paleo Diet is that it is a diet designed to closely mimic the diet we would have eaten during our evolution. You've already learned that we are designed to eat foods we would have found in the wild during this period and so it makes sense on the face of it to replace our diet with that kind of food.

However, it's important not to get too carried away with taking things literally. One common criticism of the Paleo Diet is that it doesn't really refer to a Palaeolithic diet. This complaint is rather missing the point. 'Paleo' is just a cool name; what it's really about is trying to eat more naturally and more healthily.

So if you're not getting too caught up with the specifics, you can simply apply this one very general rule to eat a Paleo-like diet:

"If a caveman couldn't eat it, neither can you."

This means that you're going to ditch the Doritos and can the soda cans. It also means – if you're being strict – no bread, no milk and no oatmeal.

Now this is where common sense needs to come in, but for now we're looking at applying a *strict* Paleo diet.

Paleos eat meats, fish, nuts, greens, vegetables, seeds, fruits and anything else they could forage or hunt. And they completely leave out the pasta, cereal and burgers.

The good news though, is that you don't actually have to hunt or forage for any of this food (though that's an option!). And actually, you shouldn't have too much problem finding these foods at all. Why? Because Paleo is super popular right now! That means you can find all kinds of organic/natural/whole food stores and any of them will provide you with all the nutritious snacks you could possibly need.

So what might a typical Paleo diet look like? Here's a typical meal plan:

Breakfast

- Scrambled egg
- Freshly squeezed orange juice

Lunch

- Tuna salad with leaves

Dinner

- Liver with sweet potato fries (fried in coconut oil) and vegetables

Dessert

- Honey nut bar

Okay, so hopefully you're starting to get the picture. The next question is whether it works, whether you should adopt it and how it can be adapted into a healthy and practical lifestyle...

Paleo Diet: The Good

Let's start by looking at the good.

And there really is a *lot* of good here.

Because what's so crucial is that you're getting a nutrient dense diet. And I mean *really* nutrient dense. Every time you eat fruit, vegetables, nuts, protein or anything else, you are getting a plethora of amino acids, vitamins, minerals and more. And as we've already discussed, the body was designed to thrive on these elements. In fact, this is what the body is actually *made* out of! We'll see later on that vitamins, minerals, amino acids and more can help to increase muscle mass, fat loss, sleep, energy... even your IQ! That's because your muscles, your brain, your metabolism – all of it is controlled and regulated by the foods we would get in our diet naturally. You're going to see more of this in the next chapters but for now, rest assured that this is *good* stuff.

Think of it like power ups in a computer game. In the wild you'd have explored the different 'levels' and found these power ups to +1 your health, +1 your strength or +1 your IQ.

Those who are really serious about eating a fully Paleo diet will often tend to consume a large amount of organ meat. The logic goes here that in the wild, this is once again what we would have eaten the most of. Think about it: if you were a primitive caveman and you just killed an antelope, you would eat the *whole thing* – you wouldn't leave the heart, the kidneys or the liver because they 'didn't look as appealing'.

And actually, this is where the densest nutrition is to be found! Eating brain provides us with tons of things like fatty acids, vitamins and minerals and amino acids. And it's amazing for *our* brains. Why? Because animal brains are made of largely the same stuff that ours are! And as organs are much more complex and important than 'foot', this is where the really good stuff goes.

Now compare this with what most of us are eating in our 'modern diet' – nothing but processed foods, sugars and other 'empty calories'. When you drink Coca-Cola, you consume just as many calories which will be stored as fat but you don't get *anything* useful that the body can use for different functions. The same goes for cakes, for burgers, for overly processed chicken nuggets, for French fries, for syrup, for pancakes... and it *especially* goes for 'low fat diet food'. Low fat diet foods actually *remove* the nutritious elements and are the equivalent of eating cardboard!

So if this is what you're living off of, then that means that your body isn't getting what it needs to thrive. Soon, you'll begin to see your skin looking less healthy, you'll feel tired and stressed, your hair might get thinner and you'll be forced to deal with brain fog.

You can keep yourself alive on nothing but chips and energy bars and soda drinks because they provide calories and a very small amount of nutrition to use as building blocks. But it's like running a car on the wrong type of fuel and your body is eventually going to start to struggle.

Perform Like a Top Athlete with Paleo

Eating a Paleo diet is a massive step in the right direction then. Eat a Paleo-like diet and you'll be consuming far fewer empty calories and you'll be getting tons of nutrition that will help your body function better in *every* regard.

And it even goes further than this. To understand just how powerful nutrition is, consider that eating organ meat will help you to get things like coenzyme Q10 and creatine. These are expensive supplements that are consumed by athletes at the highest level. They help us think sharper, burn more calories, run for longer… and you can get them entirely naturally from your diet.

Likewise, many of the nutrients you can get from a Paleo diet are things that you can buy as 'nootropics'. These are the 'smart drugs' that are being consumed by the top CEOs and investors to give them a cognitive 'edge'. But you can get *all* of this from your food.

And it makes sense! Remember: we were *designed* to eat this food.

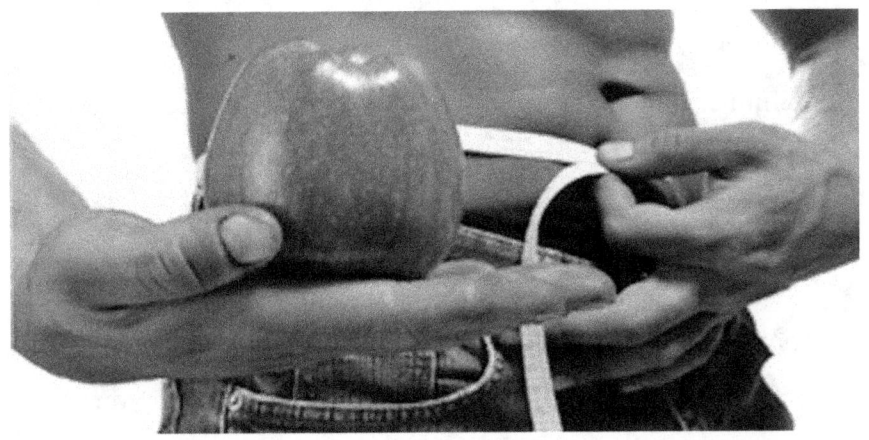

Chapter 3: The Problems With Eating a Paleo Diet

But while Paleo diets have a lot going for them, they also have a number of issues and problems.

The main problems refer simply to the fact that the Paleo diet is too reactionary.

Basically, Paleo takes a great principle and then follows it through to its extreme conclusion. This is the problem with a lot of diets and it can often lead to us eating impractical or even unhealthy diets in some cases.

Because at the end of the day, we are *not* cavemen. As much as you might wish otherwise, we do not live in caves and our environments and lifestyles are *not* the same as they were back then. A lot of this book is going to be focussed on helping you to get back to that kind of lifestyle – but unless you're incredibly committed you're not going to be living a 100% caveman lifestyle.

And even if you did: the climate has changed and so has the environment.

That's the point of evolution: we're constantly changing and constantly adapting. If you don't adapt as well, then you die. The dinosaurs learned that one!

Not all of our innovations are bad. Some of them are very good! And some of them are just *nice*.

Trying to avoid anything that is man-made just doesn't make any sense. We're going to examine vitamin tablets later and discuss how fruits and vegetables are better for you. It's true: they definitely are.

But that doesn't mean that vitamin tablets are bad for you! It doesn't mean that you can never eat vitamins in this form. And when you're in a rush, or when you're travelling, eating vitamins in that form is going to be much more practical.

Likewise, you'll probably want the occasional chocolate bar. You're not a saint! (Unless you are, in which case, I apologise.)

And not eating any bread is very likely unnecessary. The same goes for milk. In fact milk contains a ton of good nutrition and is a fantastic way to get protein.

The whole purpose of milk is to deliver crucial nutrients to young animals. This means that it is very nutrient dense. It's also a great source of saturated fats – the good kind – which can help to increase testosterone levels and brain function among other things (testosterone is made *from* cholesterol).

And there's also a problem with completely disregarding calories. Many Paleo proponents say that they like the Paleo diet because they don't need to count calories. They say that different calories effect you differently and that avoiding processed foods is enough to lead to a sudden transformation in the body.

This is true to some degree. But what's also true is that you can still get fat by eating a nutrient dense diet. In fact, it's very possible to get fat on healthy foods. And actually, the large amount of saturated fat in the Paleo diet makes it actually quite *easy* to gain weight. Fat contains 9 calories per gram, whereas carbohydrates and protein contain 4 grams of protein. By eating large amounts of saturated fat, you can potentially start eating a huge calorie surplus unintentionally which will actually lead to you gaining a lot of weight.

Let's address each of these concerns in turn…

Should You Stop Eating Bread?

Going 'gluten free' is one of the biggest health fads around right now. And it just so happens to go hand in hand with the Paleo goal of avoiding wheat and grains.

But is it necessary?

A lot of people believe that bread can have a negative impact on digestion. Celiacs and gluten-intolerant individuals are people who have an allergy to wheat and who really *should* avoid gluten. Thus gluten-free foods appeared on our shelves and companies started promoting them.

Now *everyone* is acting as though they need to avoid gluten.

In reality, only 1% of the population suffers from Celiac disease. In these individuals, gluten can cause the 'villi' to atrophy. Villi are the tiny 'fingers' that live inside the intestines and which grab onto food as it goes past to absorb nutrients. Those with Celiac disease can't eat gluten as it causes the villi to shrink away and stop working, which in turn prevents them from properly digesting and absorbing their food. The result is that they can't benefit from the nutrition in their food and they become malnourished. Symptoms include headaches, cramps, diarrhoea, tiredness and more.

Gluten sensitivity meanwhile causes similar symptoms to a lesser degree. And what's more, is that it's believed that gluten sensitivity isn't even actually *caused* by gluten but rather by something else entirely called FODMAPs.

The problem is that Celiac disease and gluten sensitivity often go undiagnosed for a long time. Because the main symptoms are depression, tiredness, headaches etc., it is often mistake for chronic fatigue syndrome, stress or even irritable bowel. Eventually, doctors suggest that patients try avoiding bread and they start to feel the best they've ever felt.

Now *lots* of find that we feel tired, groggy and stressed a lot of the time. This leads us to kind of 'hope' that we might in fact have a gluten sensitivity. If that's the case, then we should be able to avoid bread and feel better than ever. Then we avoid bread and we *convince* ourselves that's the case.

But you don't have a gluten sensitivity in all likelihood and there's no evidence that bread can negatively impact on the average individual.

What About Wheat Belly?

Another concern is something called 'wheat belly'. This is a concept that was popularized by a writer called William Davis with his book, also called *Wheat Belly*. In that book, he claimed that genetically modified proteins in bread (called gliadin) could act as an appetite stimulant through opioid channels. Davis claimed that gliadin was responsible for us eating up to 440 additional calories a day (suspiciously precise!).

He also said that starch's unique structure gave it an incredible high GI (glycemic index). This would cause bread to release its calories into the body much more quickly, resulting in a sugar high and subsequent lipogenesis (the creation of fat cells) and lethargy.

In other words, he describes bread as being the simplest of simple carbs and reacting in the body a little like pure sugar.

But here's the good news: *all* of this is wrong…

The starch in bread is exactly the same as in anything else. Starch only comes in two forms from plant tissues (amylose and amylopectin) and bread actually has a lower GI than potatoes or rice.

The stuff about gliadin is also nonsense. Gliadin only acts like an opiate in extreme high doses – higher than a human would ever eat. And research suggests that the human intestine may not absorb gliadorphin anyway.

And importantly: bread is very convenient for making sandwiches *and* very nutritious. This is an excellent source of fiber that can improve your blood pressure and circulation and it also contains a lot of minerals thanks to the added seeds.

Eat whole grain bread (not the same thing as whole wheat) and you'll get the germ, endosperm and bran from the bread. This is *very* healthy!

Sure, bread is still a relatively high GI carb. And if you eat too much of it, then you can gain weight quite easily. But there's no need to completely cut sandwiches out of your diet. It's far too complicated and far too hard to stick to. And there are no benefits.

This is a perfect example of the flaw in a lot of Paleo thinking. Just because bread wasn't around for cavemen, that doesn't mean we can't eat it. It is healthy, it is convenient and it is tasty!

Okay, What About Milk?

So that's the scoop on bread and that's why you don't need to go *that* extreme with your primal living. How about milk? Just like bread, milk is currently coming under a lot of flak from people who believe its another modern food that is causing us more harm than good.

The argument goes that milk makes you feel bad and that 60% of adults can't digest milk properly. This number is even lower for Asians and African Americans, where the percentage is said to be 5% and 25% respectively. Circumstantial evidence for milk being bad for us comes from the fact that no animal other than humans continues to consume milk post-childhood. In fact, other animals stop being able to digest milk at this age.

It's thought that this lack of digestion leads to milk not being digested. The lactose sugars then get stored in the colon where they ferment and produce cramps, bloating and nausea.

Oh dear, we should probably stop drinking milk then right?

Nope.

Because what we've just described is lactose intolerance. Yes, a percentage of people are lactose intolerant just as a percentage of people are Celiacs. If you really have lactose intolerance, then yes milk will give you diarrhoea and you'll learn that pretty early on.

That's because, at the age of 2-5, your body will stop producing lactase which is the enzyme we use to break down lactose.

BUT the rest of us *won't* stop producing that enzyme.

60% of adults can't digest milk right? Sounds like a lot! But then if you recognize that this *includes* 95% of Asians and 75% of African Americans, then you realize that *most* Caucasians *can* drink milk perfectly fine. The statistic that a lot of people don't seem to be promoting is that 90% of American adults *can* drink milk.

If you are of Asian or African decent and you're reading this, then there's a higher chance you're lactose intolerant. However, it's also highly likely that you already know that because you get frequent diarrhoea.

Another concern regarding milk is that it may drain the bones of calcium. Despite containing a lot of calcium itself, it's thought that we can't digest much of that 300mg per cup. Rather, milk acidifies the body pH and triggers a reaction. Calcium is then used to neutralize that pH and is expelled in the urine.

But here's the thing: that's probably wrong too.

This theory is largely the result of some studies including one that stated:

"Consumption of dairy products, particularly at age 20 years, was associated with an increased risk of hip fracture in old age. ("Case-Control Study of Risk Factors for Hip Fractures in the Elderly". American Journal of Epidemiology. Vol. 139, No. 5, 1994).

But let's be real for a moment here – it would be *impossible* to avoid confounding variables over such a long study. These results would have been self-reported and correlation does *not* establish causality. There were only 209 individuals in the experimental group and they were recruited from hospitals.

What's more is that all animal protein changes the blood pH in the same way that milk does. Therefore, it should all have the same effect on calcium. The only difference? Milk contains *lots* of calcium which counteracts this effect.

Also: milk doesn't only provide calcium. It also provides saturated fat, protein and carbs in equal portions and is designed to spur growth. From an evolutionary perspective, why would something we use to grow our bones, drain those same bones of calcium?

Also, also: milk is delicious. It's necessary on cereal (try it with water and see what I mean) and it's also in chocolate, tea, coffee and cheese. These are all *wonderful* things.

Even *Mark's Daily Apple*, one of the most influential blogs regarding the Paleo diet and primal living, suggests that milk is healthy and good for us overall.

Look: if you want to be 100% completely strict regarding your Paleo diet then you can be. Avoiding milk and bread won't hurt your body and the former will actually help you to eat fewer simple carbs.

But forget the idea that these things are bad for you, because there's just no evidence to support that. And I can't say that I envy you – because avoiding these foods is going to be a ton of hard work with very little reward.

Or put it another way: most of the world's top athletes and thinkers consumed both bread and milk. Somehow, neither Linford Christie nor Albert Einstein experienced the 'brain fog' or 'low energy' that naysayers are so sure they should have.

Just apply a little common sense!

Fun fact: The reason that Americans, Europeans and East Africans can drink milk is related to changes in the DNA that can be traced back several thousand years. Some suggest that the ability comes from farming in Ancient Egypt and it has even been described as one of the most modern examples of evolution in action.

If you're not lactose intolerant, then you have evolved to drink milk. So drink it!

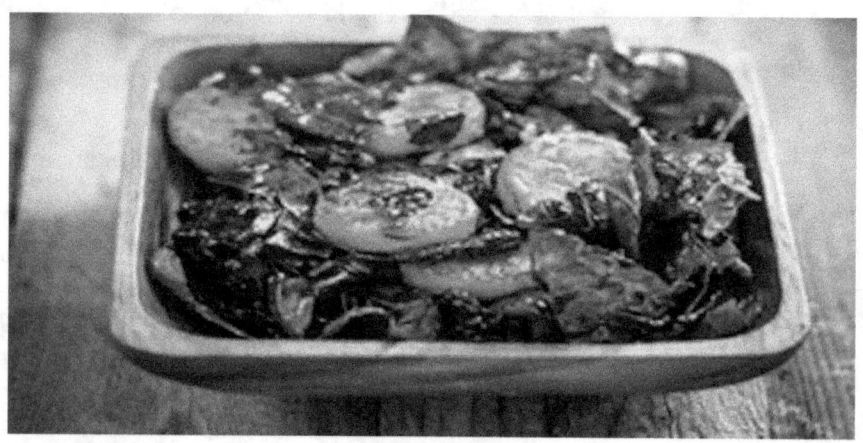

Chapter 4: How to be 'Quasi Paleo'

So the Paleo diet isn't perfect. But it does have a *lot* of good pointers.

Let's take the good and reject the bad.

The good:

- Eating more protein
- Eating organ meat

- Avoiding processed foods (on the whole – the occasional cheat won't hurt you)
- Eating a highly nutrient-dense diet

The bad:

- Believing you can completely forget about calories
- Potentially eating too much fat (related to the above point)
- Impractically avoiding milk and bread for mistaken reasons

So what you're going to do essentially is to start thinking less in a subtractive sense and more in an additive sense. If your main aim is to feel healthier, more energetic and stronger – then you should be seeking out nutrient dense foods. A pleasant side effect of this is that you'll be better satiated. Cravings are our body's way of telling us we're missing something – which is why pregnant women so often get them.

You're adding more fruits, more vegetables and more meats to your diet. Especially start trying berries and more exotic fruits (remember, we didn't evolve in the countries we live in now!) and look for nutrient goldmines - some marine plants for instance or organ meats. Smoothies – while high in sugar – are fantastic sources of vitamins and minerals and a lot of the most energetic and productive people I know *swear* by smoothies. If you're worried about the sugar, then aim for vegetable smoothies instead. Eggs are also fantastic – these are one of the only 'complete amino acid' sources, meaning that they contain all the types of protein that the human body needs. They're also high in choline, which is used to make the neurotransmitter acetylcholine. Acetylcholine is used in the brain to allow communication between neurons. Anyone who has ever experimented with 'smart drugs' will know that they're often recommended to replenish their brains with choline to avoid headaches and eggs are the best place to get this.

But nootropics can also cause damage by causing neurotransmitter imbalances. Why not just go straight for the real thing?

At the same time, you can also start avoiding things that are obviously just processed foods with no nutrients. Avoid empty calories like chocolate bars, soda drinks, ready meals and meats that have been mushed up so many times as to be unrecognizable.

Don't worry about avoiding bread and milk. You can consume less of them if you like but don't be so strict as to make this diet difficult to stick to.

Some people like the Paleo diet because it is simple and only has one easy rule.

If you're finding this all a bit complicated then, try this rule:

You can only eat foods that you could hunt, forage *or farm.*

That one extra line is going to bring us into the modern age and help make your diet LOTS more convenient.

Calories

While doing all this, you should find that you naturally start to eat healthier and this begins to reduce your snacking behaviour. You'll also naturally be getting fewer carbohydrates – while we're still eating bread, things like cake, fries and chips are out of the equation and that means you'll be consuming less sugar.

That in turn means you're going to burn more calories and this will be helped by a number of different nutrients such as l-carnitine (found in eggs among other things) that causes the body to become more efficient in burning fat.

Now we're thriving on all the things that the body is designed to thrive on but we're augmenting that with *some* healthy, modern foods like bread and milk.

BUT it's still worth keeping an eye on calories *if* your goal is weight loss. Don't consume huge amounts of fat if you're trying to lose weight because you'll be packing a ton of calories into your diet.

I'm not a fan of counting calories though and I doubt you are either. A safe way to do this then, is to try and eat a relatively consistent breakfast and lunch. This should be easy enough to do and it means you can have a very rough estimate of how many calories you'll have consumed by the time you get home in the evening.

All you now need to do is to ensure that this is significantly under your calorie goal, so that you can enjoy a nice big dinner (using only healthy, natural/farmed foods) and know it's unlikely to push you over the threshold.

I burn 2,200 calories in an average day. Thus, I have designed my lunch and breakfast to add up to around 800 calories. That means I can eat a massive dinner and as long as it's not over 1,400 calories in total, I'll be losing weight.

This is a simple, easy and *very* healthy way to eat and live.

A Little Bit About Ratios

Note that you should find that eating even a quasi-paleo diet means you are automatically consuming more protein and more saturate fat and less carbohydrates. If that's not the case, then try to tend toward it.

If you're interested in building more muscle, then try to aim for 1 gram of protein per 1 pound of bodyweight. This is the advice followed by bodybuilders and athletes and it will help you to much more easily divide up your calorie quota. Otherwise, aim to just eat *a fair amount* of protein and divide the diet roughly evenly between the three main food groups. Everything we eat, we eat for a reason. Right now, the problem is that most Americans eat far more carbohydates than anything else.

And Finally, What About Supplements?

This then brings us to one more question: how about supplements?

And the simple answer to this is: go for it!

Now of course, not all supplements are made equally and some aren't going to do much good at all. What's more, is that getting your nutrition from your diet will *always* be superior. We function better when we get vitamins and minerals this way because our body is designed to absorb them when they're presented in specific combinations. Some vitamins and minerals cancel each other out. Some are water soluble, some are fat soluble. Some take a while to enter the blood stream while others enter it immediately.

If you eat fruit, you'll get a balanced mixture of nutrients that guarantees they'll be absorbed efficiently. If you eat a multivitamin, then you *may not* get everything that's included on the label.

But then again, you'll still absorb some of it. And it's still better than nothing. So if you can get your nutrients from your diet then that's great but if you need a little extra help, then supplements can't hurt.

Likewise, protein shakes are a very convenient and healthy way to get more protein in our diet. These are simply made from whey, which is extracted from milk. Creatine is very hard to get from the diet but has a *ton* of excellent advantages for athletes and gym rats!

Again, don't throw the baby out with the bathwater! Processed foods are bad but that doesn't mean that everything 'man made' is bad!

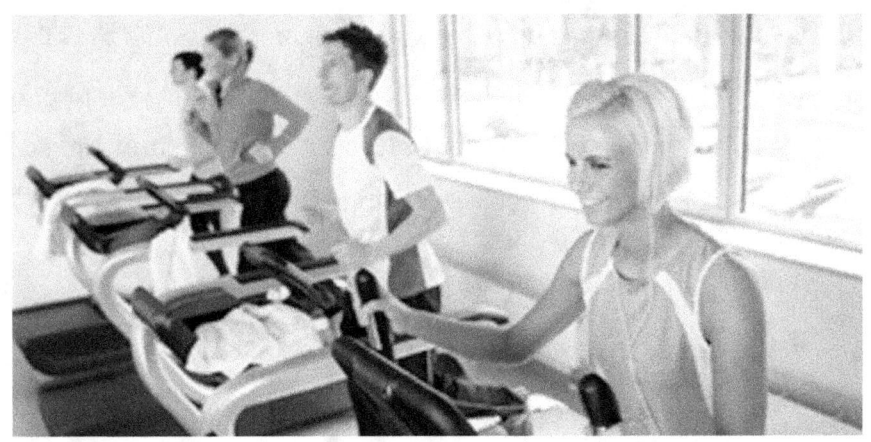

Chapter 5: Primal Exercise and Staying Active

Like I said at in chapter 1, this book is *not* a Paleo diet book. You probably guessed that already by the multiple criticisms I've levelled at the diet!

But the other way you know this isn't a Paleo book, is that I'm now going to leap into describing a ton of other aspects of 'primal living'. We've largely sorted out our diet but that's only one small part of the story.

Next up: exercise.

The Problem With Modern Exercise

Here's the problem with modern exercise:

We spend 24 hours a day, 3 days a week and 23 hours the other 4 days, doing absolutely nothing or at least very little. We may walk a little but the majority of our time is spent either sitting at a desk at work, or sitting on a sofa watching TV.

But then, for those few hours, we go absolutely crazy. After doing *nothing all day*, we suddenly throw ourselves into the gym and work like crazy for 40-60 minutes. Then we do nothing again.

What's more, is that the exercise we do is nothing like the body is used to. The exercise we do involves sitting down still and pushing against a handle. Or it involves running on a treadmill.

Even if we run in shoes on the pavement – this *isn't* what our body is designed for.

Then we go back to sitting around all day.

And we wonder why we have no energy and why it's so hard for us to get our energy levels up! And we wonder why we're still struggling to lose that weight and build muscle…

But now take a look at your cat/dog. Chances are that the story is quite different from them. They are either running around, eating, or sleeping. They very rarely will just 'sit' at all.

The same is even true in the wild. How often do you find a pigeon just sitting and watching the traffic? They are either flying around, looking for food or sleeping. They exercise *all the time* and then they lie down and recover.

Now let's take a look at our evolutionary history again. How would *we* have lived in the wild? Well, we certainly wouldn't have spent all day looking at computers. In fact, we wouldn't likely even have *sat*. We didn't have chairs and if we look at primitive man, we'll find that they would squat rather than sitting.

During the days, we would either be hunting or gathering. That would mean tracking animals long distances and for hours on end. We'd have carved stone tools, we'd have wrestled with animals and we'd have gotten into fights with other humans.

Then we'd have slept.

So in other words, we were almost always active or we were sleeping.

Before that, we would have climbed in the trees (only three million years ago we were still climbing) and primitive man would likely have climbed many craggy rocks etc.

We adapt to the lifestyle we live. If you spend all your time sitting down doing very little, then you will become efficient *at doing that*. That means that you'll find doing other more interesting things difficult and you'll be low on energy all the time.

Which means you'll never be likely to break *out* of that rat race.

Now consider how incredible you *could* be. A mountain goat is able to run across cliff faces with incredible agility and it will *never* fall. Why? Because it has been doing that its whole life and it has adapted that way. Its muscle memory is finely tuned and honed.

You could be *so much more* than you are right now.

Instead of being a fat office worker, it's time to start becoming a highly honed warrior!

Introducing Incidental Training

So the bottom line is this: our current workout programs are not enough. You can't make up for a lifetime of sitting by working out for an hour every other day.

We need to start training more throughout the day and becoming more active.

Of course that's not so easy when your boss demands that you don't do press ups on your desk. So what can you do instead?

One way to do this is with something called 'incidental' training. Or 'Nano Workouts'.

Incidental training means that you turn every day activities into a training opportunity and you make those simple things a little harder and more challenging. For instance, if you're waiting at the bus stop, why not do some calf raises on the curb?

Why not do 5 pull-ups every time you walk through the doorway that has the pull up bar installed?

And the old classic: why not take the stairs instead of the lift?

You can also multitask in order to start introducing more activity into your life. For example, when you get a call from a friend and you know it's going to be a 20 minute chat at least, why not leave the house and go for a walk?

And if you're watching TV, why not do some sit ups or some spinning at the same time?

Another tip is to take up some more active hobbies. Playing sports is a fantastic way to exercise that doesn't *feel* like work. Likewise, you could take up dance. These are rewarding, social activities that will see you burn several hundred additional calories once or twice a week.

Losing Weight Through Continuous Activity

This makes *such* a difference to your fitness, energy levels, mood and weight loss that you won't believe the changes.

A lot of people come to me for training and diet advice and often they seem very distressed at the fact that they're following all the advice – eating healthily and exercising often – but they can't lose any weight. My cousin was one such person – she couldn't lose the weight despite going to the gym three times a week and avoiding all junk food.

Meanwhile, you have my wife who never works out, who eats a lot of desert and who consistently a UK size 8.

What's the difference?

I gave them both a fitness tracker and we quickly saw the difference.

My cousin would get the tube outside her house, ride no distance down the road and then work all day. She'd then go to the gym or come home.

My wife on the other hand has a 10 minute walk this end and a 20 minute walk the other. She also *power* walks because she's very conscientious. She stands all the way on the tube (40 minutes either way) and she walks 10 minutes there and back to get her lunch.

My wife was averaging over 10,000 steps a day whereas my cousin was managing *2,000*. Meanwhile, my wife would often go for walks in the evening and we were attending a dance class at the time. And at the weekends we almost always travel somewhere to visit friends which tends to be very active too.

In short, my wife's lifestyle was just far more consistently active. She didn't choose to workout or diet but just simply by living.

Now imagine if you could start to consciously introduce much more activity throughout your day. Instead of thinking in terms of 'exercising' or 'not exercising', you're now walking, doing calf raises, doing pull ups, dancing, curling the shopping bags. Throughout the day you're burning extra calories at every opportunity and your body *will* respond!

Nano Workouts

Then you have your 'nano workouts'. These are short bursts of exercise that you can do anywhere and that will normally only require your bodyweight. It might mean that you do 50 press ups, 50 sit ups and 50 pull ups.

This is such a fast workout that it won't make you sweaty and it will be easy to convince yourself to find the time and motivation. Does it replace an in-depth workout? No – but it keeps you burning more calories throughout the day, it strengthens your heart and it even boosts your mood and energy levels. In short, this is the perfect way to 'augment' your current training program. Plus, this is an excellent 'minimum baseline'. In other words, even if you don't manage to do any other exercise that day, you'll know you've done at least this amount of training and that in turn means you'll be better off than someone who did nothing.

This trains your body to be constantly ready, to be far more energy efficient and to burn fat throughout the day. And it prevents that lethargy and staleness from setting in.

Take this excerpt from *Men's Health* that examines a study on micro workouts:

> "*If you're stuck working an 80-hour work week, Jack says that taking a few minutes every hour or so will keep your mind fresh and your body engaged. "It'll keep you mentally and emotionally sound until you can bring your activity levels up again," he says.*

> "*In fact, you can do more than minimize the damage of sitting all day, says researcher Eric Freese, Ph.D, who recently studied the benefits of sprint workouts for his dissertation at the University of Georgia. "It's possible for an athlete to maintain or even increase fitness using shorts bursts of energy," he says. Freese ran subjects through four 30-second bursts of all-out cycling sprints three days a week over a six-week period, starting at four sets and gradually increasing to eight sets. "We saw improvements across the board," Freese said. "Lowered*

triglyceride levels, increased mental energy, and improved overall mood as well."

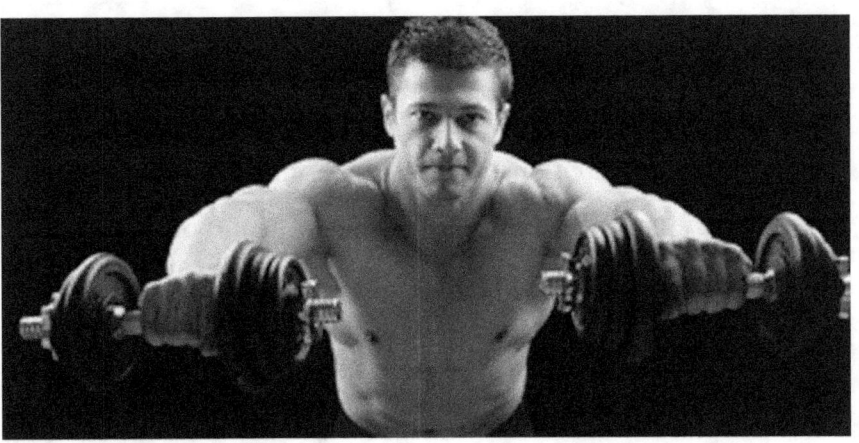

Chapter 6: Functional Training, Bodyweight Training and MovNat

The other problem is with the *way* we're working out. This is not only in terms of our overall health but also in terms of our results.

If you are training with resistance machines (like the 'chest press') then you are training in a manner that means you're sitting down and only using *one* muscle group.

Compared to lifting a rock, or climbing a tree, this is a far less efficient way to move and a far less efficient way to exercise.

These are 'compound' movements because they use the entire body. This means that the muscles have to work in unison and we develop 'functional strength' that we can actually apply in the real world without injuring ourselves.

When you use your whole body at once, it stimulates neural pathways in the brain and it helps you to burn much more fat and calories. Think about it – you're powering multiple tiny engines instead of just one! A set of press ups will get you *much* more out-of-breath than a set of press ups.

This doesn't only lead to great strength and muscle gains along with fat loss – it also helps us to move better in our lives and to feel more powerful and energetic.

Functional Strength and the 7 Primal Movements

The type of training that emphasizes compound movements to give us 'real world' strength is known as 'functional training'. The idea is that you don't curl a dumbbell because you wouldn't really use that in real life. Squatting on the other hand is something everyone should be able to do and that we can actually use in the real world. The same is true of deadlifting – which basically trains our ability to lift heavy objects off the ground.

You can actually break this down into '7 primal movements'. These are the movements that we would have needed to use in the wild and that we should all be capable of performing under stress. They are:

- Gait (walking, running etc.)
- Lunging
- Squatting
- Bending (as though picking something off the floor with legs straight)
- Torque (twisting)
- Pushing
  - Vertical push
  - Horizontal push
- Pulling
  - Vertical pull
  - Horizontal pull

What does this look like as a workout? Well, something like this:

Gait
Walking, running, dancing

Lunging
Lunge walking, lunges

Squatting
Squats, kettlebell swings, front squat

Torque (rotational chain)

Wood chopper, various oblique exercises, boxing

Bending

Straight legged deadlift, touching your toes, good mornings, leg raises

Pushing

Vertical

Press, handstand press ups

Horizontal

Bench press, chest press, press ups

Pulling

Vertical

Pull ups, chin ups, lat pull down

Horizontal

Rows, inverted press up

Now you're not just randomly build different muscles with no thought of the bigger picture. In fact, you're not focussing on the muscle at *all* but rather on the movement and on the ability that you want to gain.

This is the difference between being, slow, tired and achy with big muscles; or being a powerful, lean, coiled spring ready to strike.

And again, this is all the more reason to start supplementing your training with activities and hobbies like martial arts, yoga, dance and sports. These will help you to actually *use* your body as it was intended to be used. You'll feel lighter, faster and fuelled with energy.

Bodyweight Training and Old-Time Strongmen

I do have *some* issues with the whole 'functional strength' movement though. One of these issues is that we likely *wouldn't* have been lifting all that many barbells in the wild. And when we *did* lift something off the ground, we probably did so with useless form.

Also, gripping onto a boulder is a *lot* different from gripping onto a barbell. It helps you to develop a *lot* more strength and power in your forearms and in your grip. It also just makes you *tough* which is something you can't say of a lot of the hipsters who worry about whether or not their legs are the right distance apart before they squat.

Old-time strongmen had this right. They would train themselves to be able to do awesome things like the 'anyhow lift' which is basically a lift that lets you use *any* technique. They'd hold weights above their head with one hand while squatting and they'd lift bars that were massively thick in order to train their grip.

I'm not recommending that you do this necessarily either, as you'll find that it's a recipe for injury unless you're willing to devote a lot of time to training.

Something you *can* do though is to use bodyweight training. Things like pull ups, press ups and even rock climbing are excellent because they are functional, compound and they mimic the way we would have trained in the wild.

When you train using only your bodyweight, you will be improving your flexibility, your muscle control, your agility, your balance and more. And at the same time, you'll be able to train easily anywhere.

But what about if we merge both of these concepts together into something awesome…?

What is MovNat?

MovNat is a movement that's popular online right now. It's a portmanteaux of the words 'Movement' and 'Nature'.

And it never quite caught on the way you might expect it to. Search MovNat online and you'll see a few videos come up and a couple of articles but really not all that much.

But the few videos you *do* watch might just inspire you. These are videos of people running through the woods, doing pull ups on trees, lifting and throwing logs and climbing up rocks. It's training *in* nature and it's combining trail running with lifting weights.

And guess what? This combines functional training, with the gripping challenges of old-time strongmen and with large elements of bodyweight training.

When you do a pull up from a tree, you are forcing yourself to grab onto a thick branch that will be uneven, rough to hold and generally a lot more challenging to do pull ups from. Every branch is different and so every set of pull ups will train different muscles and challenge you in different ways.

This is just the most natural, challenging and tough workout going. And as we'll see, there are a ton of other benefits of turning your nearest woodland into your gym as well…

How much of this type of training can you realistically do? That's debatable. But on top of your usual gym workouts, your incidental training and your nano-workouts, just see if you can get a few MovNat sessions in as well.

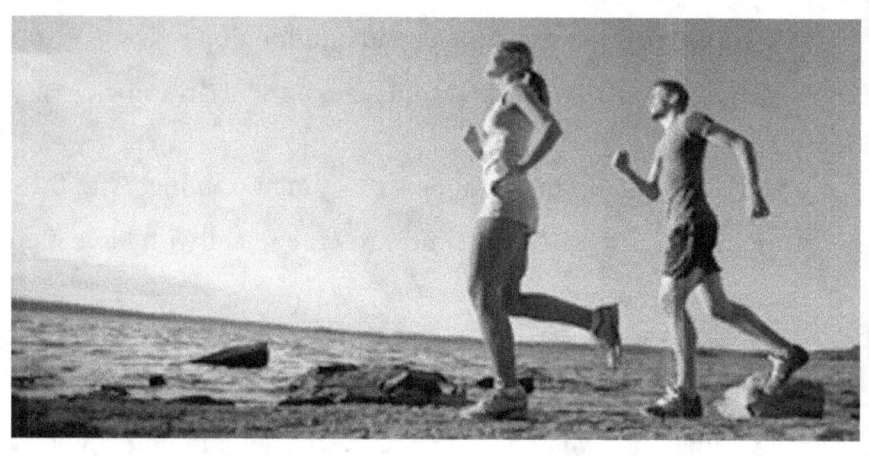

Chapter 7: On Running

The great thing about MovNat workouts is that they combine running with working out. And that running is through uneven ground which makes it 'trail running'.

And if you remember our description of how the primitive cavemen used to live, you'll recall that they spent a lot of their time tracking their prey. In fact, it's thought that our ability to keep running for long distances was our primary advantage over other animals in the wild. We weren't as fast as leopards or as strong as apes but we could follow a gazelle until it tired out and then eat it. And this is also where our brains came in so handy.

We're built to run long distances and running through the woods is a great way to do this that won't impact badly on your knees etc.

It's also 100% better than running on a treadmill. Why? Not only because you get fresh air and sun (more on that in a moment) and not only because you'll be constantly adapting to changes in the terrain (thereby training your muscles more) but also because running on a treadmill means you don't have to push forward with your feet. The floor moves underneath you, while means you only have to 'touch' the ground while remaining in place. This makes running on a treadmill significantly easier and significantly less beneficial in terms of calories burned.

Barefoot Running

Another topic that is a favorite among the primal-living crowd is the idea of barefoot running.

Once again, the theory is simple: we never evolved to run wearing shoes and as such, we shouldn't wear them when we run now. This is the central premise of books like *Born to Run* and as it happens, a lot of experts are now agreeing with the idea.

Basically, when you wear a shoe, it means your heel is padded. That means you'll likely land on the ground heel-first and in turn, this prevents your leg from cushioning the impact.

Remove your shoe and you'll be forced to land on the ball of your foot. Why? Because it allows you to bend the knee and foot more thereby absorbing the shock. This running form is known as 'chi running' or 'pose running' and it's the same method used by the Tarahumara Tribe – a tribe of indigenous humans that are known for being able to run hundreds of miles at a time.

At the same time, running without shoes means your toes are free to move around and to adapt to the terrain. When you step on a rock, your whole foot doesn't twist but rather your toes splay around it. This also uses more muscle and strengthens and toughens your feet up too.

The only problem? You've been wearing shoes your whole life. Take them off now and you'll stab your foot open on a sharp stone and damage your knees.

One option is to use a 'barefoot shoe' like the Vibram Five Fingers which fits the foot like a glove. Better yet though is to make an even more gentle transition to help avoid injury. First, head to a sports store and speak to an assistant about getting a 'minimal shoe'. This will be less padded and allow your foot to move more freely but will be something closer to the kind of footwear you're used to wearing.

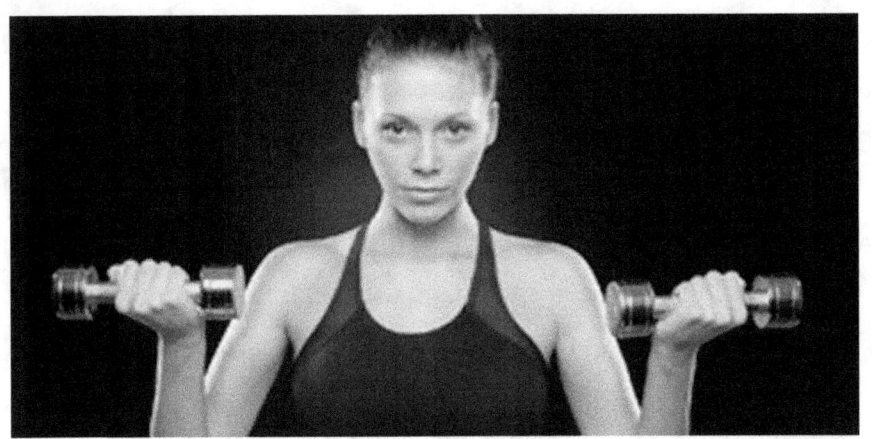

Chapter 8: Time to Un-Domesticate Yourself!

Watch some MovNat videos and feel inspired. They're swimming through rivers, jumping through dirt, climbing trees and lifting logs.

Now go and actually try to do those things and experience the reality: grazed backs, bleeding feet, freezing cold water, mud, rain… Salty water…

But before you shy away from this kind of training, just recognize that this is *kind of the point*.

What you may not realize is that you have become domesticated. Farming, shelter and technology have allowed us to become sheltered from all kinds of damage and that has resulted in our bodies becoming *soft*.

If you climb enough rocks, your hands will actually toughen up and be less prone to injury.

If you get dirty and cold, you will train your immune system and this will help you to get ill less often. Likewise, spending time in the freezing cold can encourage the release of norepinephrine which will help to increase your energy levels and focus.

Running in the cold increases your VO2 max.

Falling on unstable surfaces teaches you *not to fall next time*.

We live in soft environments and we have become soft. All we're fit for is sitting around. We're domesticated.

But if you gradually start to introduce yourself to some slightly less comfortable environments and training, then you will toughen up. And at that point, everyday life will start to feel very easy indeed.

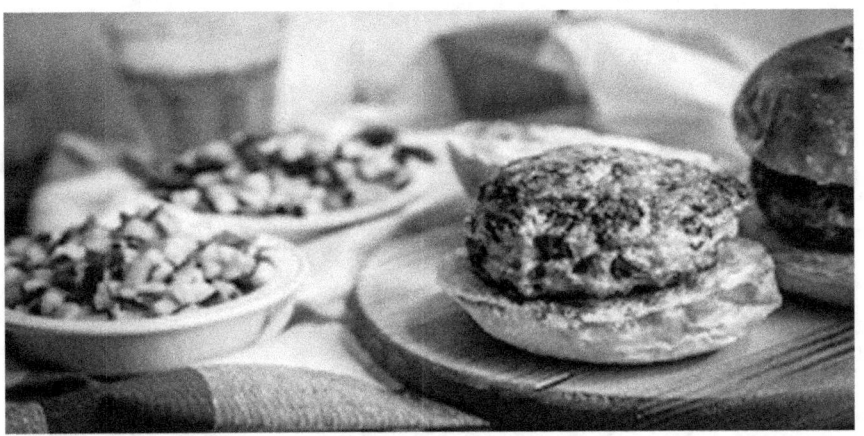

Chapter 9: The Lifestyle Habits That Are Making You Weak and Unhealthy

At this point in the book, you know how to eat more naturally and you know how to train in a way that will help you reveal your true nature.

It's exciting stuff and once you realize that you can chase that horizon, you'll find that you feel freer than you ever have done.

That's the additive stuff. But now there are also a few lifestyle changes that you need to make and a few things you need to try and *remove* from your current routines and regimes. Let's take a look:

Chronic Stress

Stress is not a bad thing. In fact, stress makes us stronger and more alert and is designed to help us escape pray, avoid danger and fight with more efficiency.

The problem is that stress isn't meant to last. In the wild, stress would have been a lion and after 30 minutes we'd either have escaped or been eaten. Today, stress means your boss hates you and this can continue for years. The result is that our body is in a constantly alert and wired state and our immune systems and digestion are constantly suppressed.

Avoiding stress is difficult of course, but you need to try and achieve it if you possibly can.

Unnatural Light

Our bodies use a combination of 'internal pacemakers' and 'external zeitgebers' in order to regulate our production of sleep hormones. To put that in plain English, we know when to sleep because of both internal and external cues.

And one of the most important of those external cues is natural light. When we detect light (which happens even with our eyes closed) our body produces cortisol and nitric oxide which helps to wake us up. When the world starts getting darker, our bodies produce melatonin which sends us to sleep.

But spend all day in an office and you've just confused your brain. Worse, if you look at a phone or computer screen in the evening, your brain will mistake that for natural sunlight and you'll produce cortisol when you're trying to sleep.

The solutions are to avoid screen time half an hour before bed and to consider investing in a daylight lamp – or leaving your curtains open and letting the sun wake you. Those latter two points can help to prevent SAD (Seasonal Affective Disorder) – a modern condition that is characterised by feelings of depression during winter. Supplementing with vitamin D in the morning may also be helpful.

Sitting

As mentioned, our bodies are not designed to sit for long periods. Sitting shortens our hip extensors, flattens our glutes and causes us to hunch forward to reach our laptop.

The result is a severe lack of flexibility which can cause all kinds of back, knee and other complaints. You can counteract this with yoga and other stretching regimes and you'd be surprised how much energy and ease of movement this can give you.

At the same time though, you should also avoid sitting as much. Try to learn to squat for comfort and consider investing in a standing desk that you can use while answering emails and doing other relatively brainless tasks.

Correct Breathing

Another problem with both stress and lots of sitting is that they cause shallow breathing. To breathe properly, sit with your back straight and chest puffed out. Breathe by letting your stomach protrude first and *then* filling up your lugs. The idea is to empty your abdominal cavity, thereby letting the diaphragm lower so that you can breathe in more oxygen by expanding your lungs.

Babies breathe this way but many of us lose this correct method of breathing as we get older. Re-learn it and you'll enjoy flatter abs, better posture and much more energy.

Cold Showers

Remember how I said earlier that the cold can wake us up *and* help us to produce more energy? Well you can do the same thing by taking one in the morning. This will wake you up, toughen you up and help you produce testosterone and norepinephrine.

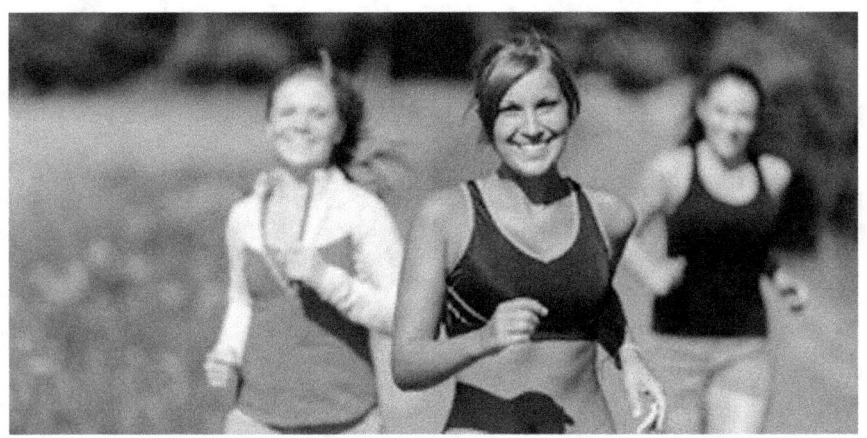

Chapter 10: Conclusion and Closing Notes

So there you have it: that's how to start living in a more primal manner. You'll be burning more fat, building more strength and toughening your body. You'll be getting more nutrition and avoiding empty calories and hunger pangs. You'll be exploring your true nature and tapping into your real potential. And at the same time, you'll feel closer to nature and enjoy all the health benefits that brings.

And there's more to this too. When you start living like this, you can actually strengthen and change your *own DNA*. This is due to something called 'epigenetics' which refers to the way that our genes express themselves. When we eat a more nutritious diet, more of our genes express themselves and this can actually get passed to our children. That should be incentive if there was none other to start living more healthily and fuelling your body the way it was designed to be.

And if you're struggling to make all these changes? Don't worry – the whole point is that you need to take it slow and give your body time to adapt.

Consider the idea of 'Kaizen' – that small, easy changes can add up to big, profound differences.

Start by adding a smoothie to your diet, maybe getting a little extra fresh air on your commute to work and perhaps doing a micro workout each morning with your bodyweight.

As you make these very minor changes, you'll find you start having more energy, more drive and better health. And this will make it easier to make all the *other* changes that will bring you closer to a natural, primal lifestyle.

The human body is always changing one way or another. If you're sitting still, then it's getting weaker. But if you start working and living and eating healthily, that means it can change for the better and you can return it to its optimal state. That's the state it was designed to be in.

Your true nature!

Healthy Living Cheat Sheet: Top Ways to Live More Naturally

You've read the ebook, you've seen the mind map and hopefully you've started applying some of these changes to your lifestyle so that you can start living healthier and more primal.

But perhaps you're still slipping up in some areas and maybe you're making a few mistakes that come with modern living. This Healthy Primal Living cheat sheet will bring you up to speed and share some of the best ways to start being healthier and getting back to your roots...

Less Screen Time!

Your body was not designed to spend all its time looking at screens. Screens trigger a stress response due partly to nature of the light they create and partly due to the need for constant concentration.

That would be bad enough but it gets a lot worse once you start introducing multiple screens and you begin and end every day with the screen.

Try introducing these few rules to start feeling fresher and less 'wired':

- No more than one screen at once
- No watching TV 'for the sake of it' – only watch when there's something you're interested in on
- No screens 30 minutes before bed – this will prevent your brain from releasing cortisol in response to what *it* thinks is sunlight. This in turn will help you to produce more melatonin and to sleep more heavily.
- No screens first thing in the morning – as soon as you check your email you'll be in a 'reactive' state of mind rather than a proactive one. Complete your 'morning routine' first.

Posture

Most of us have poor posture the vast majority of the time. This is particularly true if you sit at a desk for long hours with your shoulders hunched and your arms forward.

One quick fix for this is to tense your transverse abdominis by trying to 'pull' your navel in towards your spine. This will automatically encourage you to straighten up and will give more support for your back.

Sit Less

Better yet? Sit less.

One way to do this is by investing in a standing desk. Use this whenever you're doing a more 'mindless' task like answering emails and don't need to be highly focussed.

It's believed that in the wild, we wouldn't have sat at all and would instead have squatted. This is what you will see primitive tribes doing to this day.

Try squatting in front of the TV, standing on the bus and getting up for walks. This way, you'll avoid the stiffness and muscle shortening that can come from maintaining the same unnatural posture for long periods of time.

Take Cold Showers

Primitive man would only have been able to wash himself in the sea or in lakes – and actually this has a lot of benefits. A cold shower can help you to improve your testosterone and even your fertility (for men) while it is also great for burning calories and increasing focus by raising norepinephrine.

Best of all, cold showers are harsh. It's the last thing you want to do first thing in the morning and this takes a large amount of mental discipline and will power. This is the kind of hardiness we've lost by spending all day indoors in the warm. Time to toughen up!

Forget Bags

You know what else you wouldn't have done in the wild? Carried bags all day. If you have a shoulder bag or backpack, then you're placing unnecessary strain on your back and creating and uneven posture that your body will have to compensate for. Try to prevent this by getting bags with handles and holding them in one hand instead.

Spend Time wth Animals

Want to make your trail running even more authentic? Some people believe that primal man may have hunted alongside packs of wolves.

In his book, *The Rise of Superman*, Steven Kotler suggests that running with dogs may help us to get into a highly focussed and natural 'flow state'. I'm not sure about all that, but taking your dog for a run in the woods is a great way to reconnect with your innocent sense of fun, adventure and curiosity!

View Faces in the Morning

Seth Roberts suggests that we are happier when we see faces first thing in the morning. In the wild, we would have lived in settlements with lots of people whereas today we often live in smaller groups of 2, 3 or even one.

Hanging photos of your friends and relatives around then may help to boost your mood on an unconscious level and help you to feel a little less isolated!

Get More Sunlight

Many of us don't get enough sunlight, which leads to vitamin D deficiency and even SAD (seasonal affective disorder). To start getting more sunlight, you should create the aim of walking more. This has also been shown to improve mood and creativity – especially when we walk in natural environments.

If you can't get in more walks, consider investing in a lamp that will simulate natural daylight.

Add a Plant to Your Desk

A plant on your desk can be registered unconsciously by your brain as being subjected to a natural environment. This has been shown to help lower blood pressure and in doing so, to reduce stress and improve productivity.

Of course it also follows that sitting by a window and looking out at a garden can have even better effects!

Go Barefoot

If you're not up to barefoot running yet, try spending some time in your garden in bare feet. It's an oddly therapeutic feeling being more connected with the ground beneath you and it will help you to start developing some more strength, dexterity and feeling in your feet and toes.

Breathe Properly

Take note of how you breathe. If your chest moves first then you aren't breathing the way you're naturally designed too and you may be limiting the amount of energy your body is getting as a result. Move the abdominals first, making way for your diaphragm to drop into the cavity and let your lungs expand from the bottom.